Vegetarian Weight Loss

Jonathan Vine

Vegetarian Weight Loss

Jonathan Vine

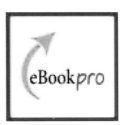

eBook-pro Publishing

Vegetarian Weight Loss\ Jonathan Vine

Editor: Hofit Carmi

ISBN-13: 978-1500663179

ISBN-10: 1500663174

Table of Contents

Introduction

One of the most popular ways for people to lose weight these days is by following a vegetarian, or vegetarian derived diet. Cutting out meat, particularly red meat makes a big improvement in your health and weight because you are cutting down the amount of bad, saturated fat you are eating and replacing it with healthier options.

Your body has less work to do fighting to digest the heavy red meat and so it can instead concentrate on looking after itself. However, whilst you may think that you will just swap your meat for the vegetarian alternatives, i.e. vegetarian burgers and so on, these can also be high in fat and other chemicals which inhibit weight loss.

If you are truly committed to losing weight on a vegetarian diet then you will need to make sure that the majority of your diet is fruits, vegetables, tofu, beans and so on, leaving the vegetarian 'meats' as a convenience food that is just occasionally eaten.

Vegetarians will avoid meat, game, fish, poultry and generally all meat by products such as animal fats and gelatine, which is found in a surprising amount of food. Vegetarians will eat a lot of fruit, vegetables, grains, beans, nuts and seeds as well as meat substitutes such as tofu and others.

There are a number of different types of vegetarians, and how extreme you go is up to you. This book will be about pure vegetarianism, though the other types are:

- Fruitarian – avoids all animal products and only eats raw foods
- Vegan – avoids all animal based foods and products too
- Lacto-vegetarian – will eat dairy products but not eggs
- Lacto-ovo-vegetarian – eats dairy and eggs

- Semi – will eat fish and / or chicken but no red meat (strictly speaking these aren't vegetarians).

A vegetarian diet is a surprisingly healthy choice for you, though you need to make sure it is a balanced diet with the right nutrients. Technically you could be a vegetarian by eating chocolate, chips and drinking sodas, but it isn't going to do your health or your waistline any good.

This book has been written to teach you everything you need to know about becoming a vegetarian and losing weight because of it. You will be surprised how easy it can be to lose weight following this diet and you don't have to worry so much about counting calories or weighing food – there is none of that going on here.

You will learn what foods to eat, what to avoid, where meat hides in every day food and how to ensure your body gets all the vitamins and minerals it needs to survive. Don't worry about protein either because you can get plenty from this diet, even as a pure vegetarian and it is easy to get additional protein if it is required.

You will learn everything you need to know about this diet and how to effectively lose weight and improve your health from it. You will be surprised by just how many health benefits the vegetarian diet has and will find out about them all in a little while. In the meantime, enjoy the book and as soon as you can, start using these delicious recipes and making your own healthy vegetarian meals.

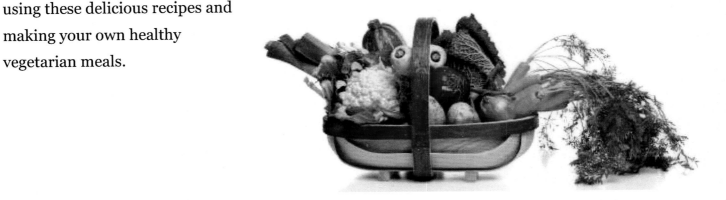

How Being Vegetarian Helps You Lose Weight

Vegetarian diets are most often much lower in sugars and fat than a meat based diet; though just cutting meat out is no guarantee of weight loss. Vegetarians are still tempted by junk food, highly processed foods and other unhealthy foods too. If you are planning on losing weight by becoming a vegetarian then you need to follow some other basic weight loss strategies to ensure you lose the weight you want.

One of the main benefits to you of the vegetarian diet is that it is lower in saturated fat (though be wary of convenience vegetarian foods which are high in these unhealthy fats) and has a higher intake of fresh fruit and vegetables. This makes a vegetarian leaner than a meat eater, so long as they are not a junk food addict.

Being a vegan means even less saturated fat as you do not eat dairy or eggs, so technically you can lose more weight. However, it is down to your personal preference, your lifestyle and your tastes. Going vegan for a few weeks can help kick start your weight loss.

Just stopping eating meat isn't going to help you lose weight if you are still consuming huge amounts of calories every day. You will need to discipline yourself and control your calorie intake like you would on any diet. However, remember that vegetables in particular are low in calories and most diets instruct you to "pile 'em high" on your plate!

Just watch your portion sizes, particularly with the more fattening foods that you eat; the same goes for restaurants. Prepare your meals in advance and plan what you are going to eat and you will find it much easier to lose weight. Also make sure you have some healthy, low fat snacks around so you are less likely to reach for a candy bar.

Try to avoid frying food when you can and bake, steam or grill instead because it is lower in fat and much healthier for you.

In order to lose weight reliably you will need to increase your exercise levels to burn fat and excess calories. Regular cardio and weight training will help to improve your health and help you process food better. You can lose some weight as a vegetarian but to really turbo-charge your weight loss you need to incorporate exercise into your daily regime. Join a gym, get a personal trainer and start working out because you will find your weight loss speeds up and that you lose inches as you start to firm up your muscles.

The main component of your diet will be vegetables and fruits, together with beans and whole grains. With all meats and fish eliminated from your diet you are already eating many of the foods that are recommended by diet plans to help you lose weight. Studies have shown that a low fat vegan diet alone will help you to lose 1lb a week without including exercise or any other factors!

Be aware though that if you are loading up on pasta, cereal and breads (high carbohydrate / low nutrition) then you will struggle to lose weight. Eating too many sugary foods or the meat substitutes is also going to contribute to you not losing weight. Remember that by applying these principles to your vegetarian diet you will speed up your weight loss and improve your health further.

Vegetarianism vs. Veganism

We have touched on some of the different types of vegetarianism that there are. The two main approaches are either veganism or vegetarianism.

A vegan will eliminate all meat products from their diet including eggs, dairy and gelatine. Typically a vegan will avoid any products that are made from animals such as leather, wool, down, silk and so on. Many vegans choose to follow this lifestyle because they have care deeply for animals and the environment.

Vegetarians however will wear leather, wool and silk and many will eat eggs and dairy products. Most vegetarians will avoid products that contain gelatine though some will quietly ignore it as it is in such a tiny quantity. It is your choice which you follow at the end of the day.

Nutritionally there is not a huge amount of difference between a pure vegetarian and a vegan; the latter will need a vitamin B12 supplement. A lacto-ovo vegetarian should not need this supplement as they will get it from eggs and dairy.

For those that choose the vegan approach it is usually related to their love and respect for animals. From a weight loss point of view, a vegan diet can help to kick-start your weight loss and help you lose an extra couple of pounds when you need it.

Whether you start off as a vegetarian and do weeks of vegan eating or what type of vegetarian diet you choose to follow is entirely up to you. Make sure you have thought through all the different options and selected the right type of diet for you.

The Health Benefits Of The Vegetarian Diet

Whilst the vegetarian diet is going to help you to lose weight, it is also going to help to improve your health. A lot of research has been performed in to the benefits of vegetarianism, and the result is the federal government even recommend that the majority of your daily calories come from vegetables, fruits and grain products.

It is estimated that around 70% of all diseases, including a third of all cancers are caused by diet! Vegetarians have a lower risk of obesity, high blood pressure, diabetes, coronary artery disease and cancers including prostate, stomach, breast, oesophageal and colon cancer. You can already see the benefits of cutting out meat!

You will be interested in knowing that vegetarians are typically healthier than the average American, particularly when it comes to reversing heart disease and reducing the risks of cancers. A low fat vegetarian diet has been proven to be the best way to stop coronary artery disease progressing or to prevent it.

Every year, over a million people in American die from cardiovascular disease; it's the number one killer in the USA. However, the mortality rate from this disease is significantly lower in vegetarians due to the lower cholesterol levels and that you consume less saturated fat. A vegetarian will consume more anti-oxidants, more fiber and more vitamins and minerals.

The standard Western diet is high in processed foods full of chemicals, sugar and salt and low in plant based foods. This diet is actually killing us all slower. The obesity statistics are shocking and the associated health problems even worse.

Between the years of 1986 and 1992 the Preventive Medicine Research Institute in Sausalito California conducted a study in to the vegetarian diet. They discovered that an overweight person who ate a low fat vegetarian diet lost, on average, twenty four pounds in year one and in five year's time had still kept the weight off. This weight was lost without feeling hungry, measuring portions or counting calories.

Studies have also shown that a vegetarian diet will extend your life by around thirteen years of good health! Meat eaters will typically not only have a shorter lifespan but will also suffer from more disabilities at the end of their lives. Studies have also shown that meat eaters also experience sexual and cognitive dysfunction at a younger age.

The vegetarian diet is packed full of vital nutrients such as calcium, magnesium, phosphorus, vitamin D and more, all of which are vital to your health and wellbeing. These vitamins contribute to a healthier, longer diet. If you choose not to eat dairy then you can get your minerals and vitamins from tofu, soymilk, dry beans, broccoli, collard greens, kale and so on.

A fringe benefit of vegetarianism is that your risk of food borne illness is dramatically reduced. According to CDC statistics there are 76,000,000 food borne illnesses each year across the United States. The majority of these illnesses come from meat and seafood!

The vegetarian diet also eases the symptoms of the menopause, particularly as soy is the best natural source of phytoestrogens, but they are also found in many other vegetables too. As women often gain weight during the menopause as their metabolism slows down, a low fat vegetarian diet can help keep the extra pounds off.

Another advantage of the vegetarian diet is that your energy levels increase. As you are not spending so much of your energy digesting heavy foods. The foods you eat as a vegetarian tend to be more nutritious, meaning your body has the vitamins it needs to be healthy.

A good, balanced vegetarian diet is free from the saturated fats that clog up your arteries and restricts the oxygen supply to your body. Your diet will also be high in complex carbohydrates which give you more energy that lasts longer.

Vegetarians also help the environment with meat production causing deforestation, global warming and more. According to the EPA in the USA, animal and chemical waste runoff from factory farming causes over 173,000 miles of polluted streams and rivers.

Many of the toxins a human eats come from meat and seafood, with fish in particular storing heaving metals and carcinogens that cannot be removed. Many meat and dairy products also have high levels of growth hormones, steroids and antibiotics which are taken in to your body.

Around 70% of the grain produced in the USA is fed to animals. There are around seven billion livestock animals in the United States which consume five times more grain than the American population itself. The grain fed to animals is worth about $80 billion on the export market and would feed around 800 million people!

Every year over ten billion animals are slaughtered for human consumption, which is a major factor for many vegetarians in giving up meat. That and the treatment of animals – factory farming, force feeding, poor conditions and so on. What you may not realize is that state laws on animal cruelty specifically exclude farm animals from even the most basic, humane protection.

Being a vegetarian is cheaper, particular if you don't rely on the expensive textured vegetable protein used as a meat substitute. Around 10% of the average American's income is spent on meat. By cutting out the meat, on average, you could save around $4,000 a year!

The vegetarian's dinner plate is always full of color, which means they are full of vital vitamins and minerals. Yellow and orange foods are high in carotenoids, as are leafy green vegetables, which are also high in chlorophyll. Red and purple foods are high in anthocyanins. These are both important for your health and will help boost your immune system.

With so many personal and environmental benefits to being a vegetarian your plan to lose weight suddenly seems even more appealing. You will notice that as you lose weight you feel healthier, have more energy and are able to enjoy life more because of it.

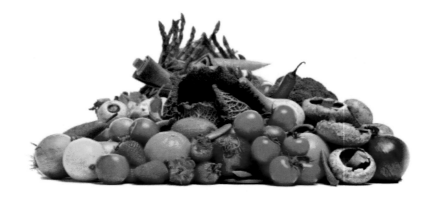

Foods To Eat And Foods To Avoid

As a vegetarian you will avoid all meat and seafood products, though some will eat eggs and dairy. On top of this there are a lot of other things that a vegetarian can eat and this chapter is designed to help you understand how the vegetarian diet works and what foods you can eat and enjoy.

Grains

Grains are an important part of the vegetarian diet and it is recommended that you eat between five and seven servings per day, of which half should be whole grains. Grains include oats, barley, wheat, rice, bread and pasta, many of which are now fortified with vitamins such as zinc, iron and vitamin B-12 which are more commonly found in meat and seafood.

Proteins

Non-vegetarians get their protein from meat, but you will need to get your protein from other sources including beans, legumes, soy and nuts. For those who eat it, dairy and eggs are a good source of protein too. Iron normally comes from meat but instead you can find it in dry beans, lentils, soybeans, tofu, peas and spinach. Remember to consume foods rich in vitamin C at the same time as they help you absorb iron.

Fruits And Vegetables

Fruits and vegetables are consumed in large amounts by a vegetarian. Whether these are fresh or frozen is entirely up to you, but whichever you choose they are high in vitamins and minerals. You want between six and eight servings of vegetables every day and three or four of fruit. If you are not eating eggs or dairy then make sure you eat plenty of dark green leafy vegetables as they are high in nutrients your body needs.

Fats

We are taught that low fat diets are good for us, but your diet needs to be low in saturated fats. The proper fats are important for the operation of your body and you need around two servings per day. You need fats that are high in Omega-3 fatty acids which you can get from an ounce of nuts or seeds, a teaspoon of olive oil or two tablespoons of nut butter.

As a vegetarian you will be eating plenty of nutrient dense foods though because of the lack of meat, particularly if you are avoiding dairy and eggs, you may need to take some supplements to ensure you are getting the right nutrients. See the chapter late in this book to understand this more.

Foods To Be Careful Of

As a vegetarian you will need to be careful about some of the foods you are eating because meat does creep into rather a lot of foods. This section will help you understand what foods you need to watch out for.

Soups are delicious and great for a vegetarian, but be careful when dining out or buying cans of soup as often they will be made with a chicken, beef or fish base. Make sure you ask in a restaurant and read the ingredients on the can just to be sure, but it is easy to make your own delicious soups at home!

A lot of salad dressings in restaurants are built on bacon fat and Caesar dressing contains anchovies. Make sure you check the ingredients in the dressing to make sure it is vegetarian friendly and doesn't have an animal hiding in it.

Cheese is eaten by some vegetarians but not all cheese is vegetarian! Some cheeses use animal rennet in their manufacturing, which is enzymes from animal stomachs! You will find cheeses that are vegetarian or you can ignore this fact, it is up to you. If you check the labels you will find the vegetarian cheeses are labelled as such.

If you eat tortillas then check the ingredients as many of them are made with animal products, as are many other chips. Some of the meaty flavors of chip are in fact vegetarian and typically they will be labelled so you know what you can and cannot eat.

Look out for gummy type sweets as well as usually these will contain gelatine which comes from animal bones. There are some vegetarian versions if you are being strict, though a lot of vegetarians will overlook this fact in their need for candy! Check the ingredients of Jello and marshmallows as these can also contain gelatine.

And bad news for many men here, some beers aren't entirely vegetarian as they can be clarified with something called isinglass or fish bladders. Some beers are fine, though it is up to you how strict you want to be here.

There are a lot of foods that you may think are safe to eat but are in fact not vegetarian. Take some time to read the labels and you will soon work out which foods you can and cannot eat following the above guidelines.

Vegetarian Sources Of Vitamins And Protein

We've touched on the need for proper nutrition previously in this book and this chapter is dedicated to helping you understand how you can ensure you get the right levels of nutrition from the foods you are eating. This is very important for new vegetarians to ensure you do not become deficient in any vitamins or minerals which could harm your health.

A vegetarian who doesn't eat the right type of diet could end up with chronic fatigue and a compromised immune system so it is important that you eat the right types of food.

Firstly you need to decide what type of vegetarian diet you are going to follow. A lacto-ovo vegetarian is going to get a lot more essential nutrients than a pure vegan, but you can still be healthy when following the latter diet.

You need to understand the vitamin content of food and ensure that you eat a balanced diet that includes plenty of fruit and vegetables, as these are your primary sources of vitamins. You want around six to eight portions of vegetables and three to four of fruit every single day. If you are not getting these then you are going to become deficient in vital nutrients.

Protein is essential and it isn't hard to get the required levels on a vegetarian diet. However, you need to make sure it is coming from good sources such as tofu, beans, lentils, chickpeas and so on. You can get protein from textured vegetable proteins (meat replacements) though this is highly processed and can contain chemicals, saturated fats and other unwanted additives.

You can also get your protein from whole grains and leafy green vegetables as well as dairy products and eggs. If you are concerned about your protein levels then you can use vegetarian protein powders mixed into smoothies or juices.

If you feel that you are lacking in the proper nutrition then get some vitamin tablets and start taking them. You may find you are not getting enough vitamin B-12, calcium and iron but you can get iron from mushrooms, tofu and cashew nuts. If you do choose to take an iron supplement then you will need to also take a vitamin C supplement to help you absorb the iron.

Calcium is found in the leafy green vegetables as well as fortified products such as soy milk and so on. If you are taking a calcium supplement then also take a vitamin D supplement as this will help you absorb the calcium properly.

B-12 is the big problem for pure vegans because it is found in animal products and not in vegetables. However, you can get this from fortified yeasts, cereal or soy milk. It is found in eggs and dairy products if you are a lacto-ovo vegetarian.

You will also need Omega-3 fatty acids which are vital for your brain development, eyesight and muscles. This is found in eggs but can also be found in pure vegetarian sources such as soybeans, tofu, walnuts, flaxseed oil and canola oil. If you are in doubt about how much of this you are getting then take a supplement.

When you are getting the right nutrition from your vegetarian diet you will feel fantastic and really benefit from following this way of eating. Make sure you are getting all the right vitamins and if you feel you aren't then take some supplements to give your system a boost.

Vegetarian Weight Loss Recipes

This section is all about giving you some delicious recipes, which you can use to make great food at home. Some of these will be pure vegetarian, and some lacto-ovo vegetarian. Choose the meals you want to make and enjoy making them. You can have lots of fun building on these recipes and experimenting with them.

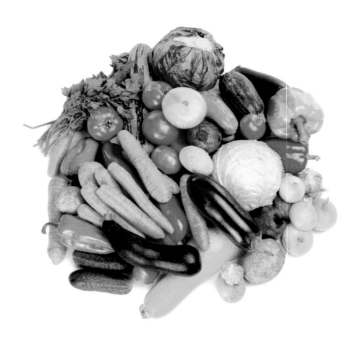

Vegetarian Breakfasts

Breakfast is an important meal and you need suitable levels of protein and nutrition in order to kick-start your metabolism for the day. People who skip breakfast will find their metabolism slows for the day, meaning less weight loss and more calories converted to fat! Try these delicious recipes, many of which can be made in advance.

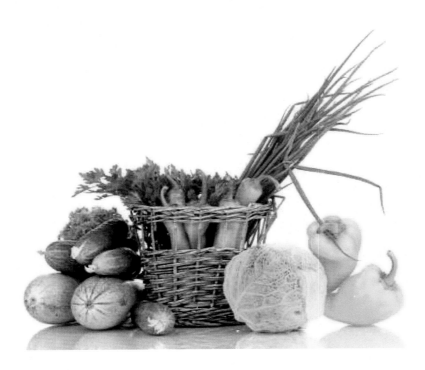

Scrambled Egg Burritos

Serves 4.

Time to make: 30 minutes

Ingredients:

- **4 whole wheat flour tortillas (9 inch diameter)**
- **4 large eggs**
- **2 cups salsa**
- **½ cup grated vegetarian Cheddar or Pepper Jack cheese**
- **¼ cup low fat sour cream**
- **4oz can of chopped green chillies**
- *1 teaspoon extra-virgin olive oil*
- *Salt / pepper to taste*

Method:

1

Preheat your oven to 350F.

2

Wrap the tortillas in tin foil and warm for five to ten minutes in the oven.

3

Mix the eggs with the salt and pepper in a bowl until well blended.

4

Heat the oil in a non-stick pan.

5

Cook the chillies for a minute before adding the eggs. Continue to cook for another one to three minutes (depending on desired consistency) stirring slowly throughout.

6

Divide the eggs between the tortillas, sprinkle a couple of tablespoons of cheese over each one and roll up.

7

Serve immediately with sour cream and salsa

Raspberry Almond Oatmeal

Serves: 4

Time to make: 15 minutes

Ingredients:

- ½ cup rolled oats
- 1 cup almond milk
- ½ cup water
- 2 tablespoons flax seeds, ground
- 1 ripe banana, mashed
- 2 tablespoons maple syrup
- ½ cup fresh raspberries
- 2 tablespoons sliced almonds

Method:

1

In a saucepan, combine the almond milk with the water and bring to a boil.

2

Stir in the rolled oats, banana and flax seeds and cook for 5-8 minutes on low heat until thick and creamy.

3

Remove from heat and stir in the maple syrup.

4

Spoon the mixture in 2 serving bowls and top with fresh raspberries and sliced almonds.

Soy Pocket Eggs

Serves 4.

Time to make: 15 minutes

Ingredients:

- 4 eggs
- **4 teaspoons canola oil**
- **2 tablespoons low salt soy sauce**
- **1 tablespoon minced scallion greens**
- **1 tablespoon dried basil**
- **2 teaspoons black sesame seeds**
- **1½ teaspoons rice vinegar**
- **1 teaspoon toasted sesame oil**
- **¼ teaspoon ground white pepper**

Method:

1

Mix the sesame oil, vinegar, scallion greens and soy sauce in a small bowl and put to one side.

2

Heat the canola oil in a non-stick pan and ensure the pan is well coated with oil.

3

Crack two eggs into one small bowl and the other two eggs into another small bowl.

4

Quickly pour two eggs on to one side of the pan and the other two on to the other side, allowing the egg whites to flow together to produce a large piece.

5

Sprinkle the pepper, basil and sesame seeds over the eggs and cook until the whites are brown on the bottom and crispy at the edges (about three minutes).

6

Keeping it in one piece, flip the eggs and cook for another minute or two on the other side until the whites are crispy and brown.

7

Pour the sauce over the eggs, simmering for 30 seconds on each side.

8

Cut in to wedges to serve and drizzle the remaining sauce from the pan over the eggs.

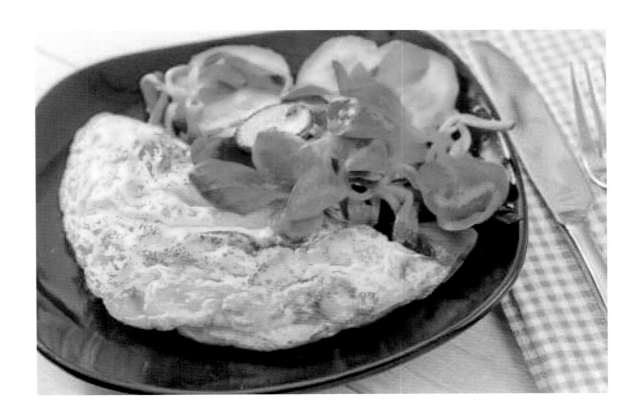

Cheddar Spinach Quiche

Serves: 8

Time to make: 1 hour 15 minutes

Ingredients:

Crust:
- 2 cups all-purpose flour
- 1 pinch salt
- ½ teaspoon baking powder
- ½ cup cold butter, cubed
- 2-4 tablespoons cold water

Filling:
- 5 eggs
- 1 cup heavy cream
- 2 tablespoons olive oil
- 3 cups fresh spinach, shredded
- 2 garlic cloves, chopped
- 1 shallot, chopped
- Salt, pepper to taste
- 1 ½ cups Cheddar cheese, grated

Method:

1

To make the crust, mix the flour with the salt and baking powder.

2

Stir in the cold butter and rub it into the flour until the mixture looks sandy.

3

Pour in the cold water, 1 tablespoon at a time and mix until it comes together into an easy to make dough.

4

Place the dough on a well-floured working surface and roll it into a 1/4-inch thick sheet. Transfer the dough into a pie or tart pan and press it well on the sides and bottom of the pan. Place the pan in the freezer until you make the filling.

5

For the filling, heat the olive oil in a skillet and stir in the garlic and shallot. Sauté for 5 minutes.

6

Stir in the shredded spinach and sauté for 5 minutes just until soft. Remove from heat and let it cool down.

7

In a bowl, mix the eggs with the heavy cream. Add salt and pepper to taste, then stir in the spinach mixture and half of the grated Cheddar.

8

Pour the filling into the crust and top with the remaining cheese.

9

Bake in the preheated oven at 350F for 40-50 minutes or until the edges and top turn golden brown.

10

Serve it slightly warm or chilled.

Avocado Banana Smoothie

Serves: 4

Time to make: 15 minutes

Ingredients:

- **1 ripe banana, mashed**
- **1 ripe avocado, peeled**
- **2 cups almond milk**
- **4 dates, pitted**
- **2 tablespoons chia seeds**
- **2 tablespoons maple syrup**
- **1 pinch cinnamon powder**

Method:

1

Combine all the ingredients in a blender and pulse until the smoothie is well blended.

2

Pour the smoothie in your favorite glasses and serve it fresh because it tends to change color in time.

Banana Walnut Bread

Serves: 12

Time to make: 50 minutes

Ingredients:

- **1 cup all-purpose flour**
- **½ cup coconut flour**
- **1 teaspoon baking soda**
- **1 teaspoon baking powder**
- **1 pinch salt**
- **½ teaspoon cinnamon powder**
- **½ teaspoon ground cardamom**
- **1 pinch nutmeg**
- **1 cup dates, pitted**
- **¼ cup maple syrup**
- **½ cup vegetable oil**
- **4 eggs**
- **3 ripe bananas, mashed**
- **1 cup walnuts, chopped**

Method:

1

In a large bowl, sift the flours with the salt, baking powder, baking soda, cinnamon, cardamom and nutmeg.

2

In a blender or food processor, combine the dates with the eggs, maple syrup and vegetable oil. Pulse until smooth and well blended.

3

Pour this mixture over the flour. Mix well then stir in the mashed bananas and chopped walnuts.

4

Pour the batter in a loaf pan lined with parchment paper and bake in the preheated oven at 350F for 40-45 minutes or until golden brown.

5

Let it cool in the pan before serving.

Red Pepper and Artichoke Frittata

Serves 2.

Time to make: 35 minutes

Ingredients:

- **4 eggs**
- **14oz can of artichoke hearts (rinsed and coarsely chopped)**
- **2 minced garlic cloves**
- **1 diced red bell pepper**
- **2 teaspoons extra-virgin olive oil (divided)**
- **¼ cup grated Parmesan cheese**
- **1 teaspoon dried oregano**
- **¼ teaspoon crushed red pepper**
- **Salt / pepper to taste**

Method:

1

Heat a teaspoon of oil in a non-stick pan.

2

Cook the bell pepper for around two minutes until tender.

3

Add the crushed red pepper and garlic and cook for a further half a minute before transferring to a plate. Wipe out the pan.

4

Whisk the eggs in a bowl and stir in the Parmesan, artichoke hearts, bell pepper mixture and oregano. Season with salt and pepper to taste.

5

Set a rack around four inches from the heat source and preheat your broiler.

6

Brush the pan with a teaspoon of oil and heat.

7

Pour the egg mixture in and tilt to ensure it is evenly distributed.

8

Reduce the heat and cook until the bottom is a golden color, lifting the edges to all the uncooked egg to flow underneath (around 4 minutes).

9

Then put the pan in the broiler for another couple of minutes until the top is set.

10

Slide the frittata on to a plate, cut into wedges and serve immediately.

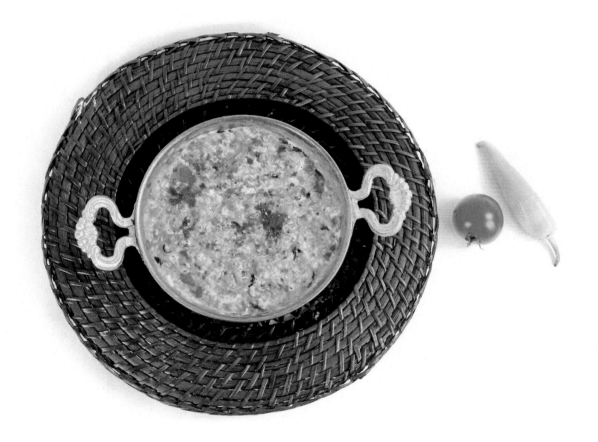

Onion and Herb Frittata

Serves 1.

Time to make: 10 minutes

Ingredients:

- **1 cup diced onion**
- **2 tablespoons reduced fat ricotta cheese**
- **2 teaspoons chopped fresh herbs**
- **½ cup of liquid egg substitute**
- **¼ cup plus 1 tablespoon of water (divided)**
- **1 teaspoon extra-virgin olive oil**
- **Salt / pepper to taste**

Method:

1

Boil the onion and the quarter cup of water in a non-stick pan. Cover and cook until the onion starts to soften (around two minutes). Uncover and cook for another couple of minutes until the water has evaporated.

2

Drizzle in the oil and stir until coated.

3

Cook for another two minutes, stirring regularly, until the onion has started to brown.

4

Pour in the egg substitute and cook, stirring constantly, for about twenty seconds until the egg starts to set.

5

Continue cooking, lifting the edges so the uncooked mixture flows underneath and the egg is mostly set – about another thirty seconds.

6

Reduce the heat, sprinkle the herbs over the frittata and season to taste.

7

Spoon the cheese over the top of the frittata.

8

Lift the edge of it up and drizzle the last tablespoon of water underneath it.

9

Cover and cook until the egg is set and the cheese is hot (around two minutes).

10

Slice the frittata from the pan on to a plate and serve.

Waffles with Cherry Sauce

Serves 6 (each serving is one waffle and ¼ cup of sauce)

Time to make: 1 hour

Cherry Sauce Ingredients:

- 2 cups of fresh pitted cherries (frozen is fine but do not thaw them)
- ¼ cup each of water and honey
- 2 teaspoons corn-starch
- 1 teaspoon vanilla extract
- 1 teaspoon lemon juice

Waffle Ingredients:

- 2 cups whole wheat flour (white)
- 2 large eggs
- 2 cups low fat buttermilk
- ½ cup fine cornmeal
- ¼ cup light brown sugar (packed)
- 1 tablespoon canola oil / extra-virgin olive oil
- 2 teaspoons vanilla extract
- 1½ teaspoons baking powder
- ½ teaspoon baking soda
- ¼ teaspoon salt

Method:

1

Mix all the sauce ingredients in a pan and bring to the boil. Cook for about a minute, stirring occasionally until it thickens. Put the mixture to one side whilst you make the waffles.

2

Preheat your oven to 200F and put a baking sheet on the middle rack.

3

Whisk the flour together with the baking powder, cornmeal, baking soda and salt in a large bowl.

4

In a separate bowl mix beat the eggs with the brown sugar.

5

Add the oil, vanilla and buttermilk and whisk until well mixed.

6

Add the wet ingredients to the bowl with the dry ingredients and stir until combined.

7

a Belgian waffle iron and coat it lightly with cooking spray.

8

Add enough butter to cover a third of its surface and distribute evenly with a spatula.

9

Close the waffle iron and cook for between four and five minutes until golden brown.

10

Transfer the cooked waffles to the baking tray to keep warm (do not stack) until you have finished making the whole batch of waffles – use more cooking spray as required.

11

Warm the sauce and serve it poured over the waffles.

Flaxseed Banana Muffins

Serves: 18

Time to make: 35 minutes

Ingredients:

- **¼ cup flax seeds, ground**
- **1 cup all-purpose flour**
- **1 cup whole wheat flour**
- **1 teaspoon baking soda**
- **1 pinch salt**
- **1 teaspoon cinnamon powder**
- **1 cup shredded coconut**
- **3 ripe bananas, mashed**
- **¼ cup coconut oil**
- **1 cup water**
- **¼ cup maple syrup**

Method:

1

In a bowl, combine the flax seeds with the flours, baking soda, salt, cinnamon and shredded coconut.

2

In a different bowl, mix the bananas with the coconut oil, water and maple syrup. Pour this mixture over the dry ingredients and mix very well.

3

Spoon the batter into your muffin cups lined with muffin papers and bake them in the preheated oven at 350F for 25 minutes or until golden brown and fragrant.

4

Let them cool in the pan before serving.

Cranberry Muesli

Serves 2

Time to make: 10 minutes (plus overnight chilling time)

Ingredients:
- 6 tablespoons rolled oats (not steel cut or quick cooking)
- 2 tablespoons dried cranberries
- ½ cup low fat plain yoghurt
- ½ cup cranberry juice (either unsweetened or sweetened with fruit juice)
- 1 tablespoon sunflower seeds (unsalted)
- 1
- tablespoon wheat germ
- 2 teaspoons honey
- ¼ teaspoon vanilla extract
- Dash of salt

Method:
Mix everything in a bowl, cover and refrigerate overnight (between 8 hours and one day).
Serve as is or with soy / cow / almond milk.

Coconut Chia Pudding

Serves: 4

Time to make: 10 minutes

Ingredients:
- 2 cups coconut milk
- 4 tablespoons chia seeds
- 4 tablespoons shredded coconut
- 2 tablespoons maple syrup
- 1 pinch cinnamon powder
- ½ teaspoon vanilla extract
- ½ mango sliced (or raspberry)

Method:

1

Mix the coconut milk with the chia seeds, shredded coconut, maple syrup, cinnamon and vanilla in a bowl.

2

Cover the bowl with plastic wrap and let it soak for 3 hour or even overnight.

3

Top it with sliced mango just before serving.

Breakfast Granola

Serves: 10

Time to make: 40 minutes

Ingredients:

- **3 cups rolled oats**
- **1 cup coconut flakes**
- **1 cup pecans, chopped**
- **½ cup sliced almonds**
- **¼ cup pumpkin seeds**
- **¼ cup sunflower seeds**
- **¼ cup chia seeds**
- **1 teaspoon cinnamon powder**
- **1 pinch salt**
- **¼ cup maple syrup**
- **½ cup coconut oil**

Method:

1

Combine all the dry ingredients in a bowl and set aside.

2

In a small saucepan, mix the maple syrup with the coconut oil and melt them together over low heat. Pour this mixture over the dry mixture and mix gently.

3

Spread the granola in a baking tray lined with parchment paper and bake in the preheated oven at 330F for 30-35 minutes.

4

When done, let the granola cool in the pan then store in an airtight container.

Cranberry and Lemon Muffins

Makes 12 muffins

Time to make: 1 hour

Ingredients:

- 1 egg
- ¾ cup non-fat plain yoghurt
- ½ cup and 2 tablespoons sugar (divided)
- A third of a cup of canola oil
- 1½ cups white whole wheat flour
- ½ cup fine cornmeal
- 1½ cups of coarsely chopped cranberries (fresh or thawed)
- 3 teaspoons grated lemon zest (divided)
- 2 tablespoons lemon juice
- 2 teaspoons baking powder
- 1 teaspoon baking powder
- 1 teaspoon vanilla extract
- ¼ teaspoon salt

Method:

1

Preheat your oven to 400F.

2

Fill a muffin tray with paper muffin liners.

3

Whisk the egg, oil, yogurt, half a cup of sugar, lemon juice, two teaspoons lemon zest and the vanilla extract in a bowl.

4

Whisk the salt, baking soda, cornmeal, baking powder and flour in a large bowl.

5

Add the yoghurt mixture to the flour mixture and fold until it is almost blended.

6

Fold in the cranberries gently.

7

Divide the mixture between the muffin cups.

8

Mix the remaining teaspoon of lemon zest and two tablespoons of sugar in a bowl. Sprinkle this over the top of the muffins.

9

Bake the muffins for 20 to 25 minutes until golden brown and they spring back when you touch them.

10

Let them cool for ten minutes before transferring them to a wire rack.

11

Allow them to cool for another five minutes before eating.

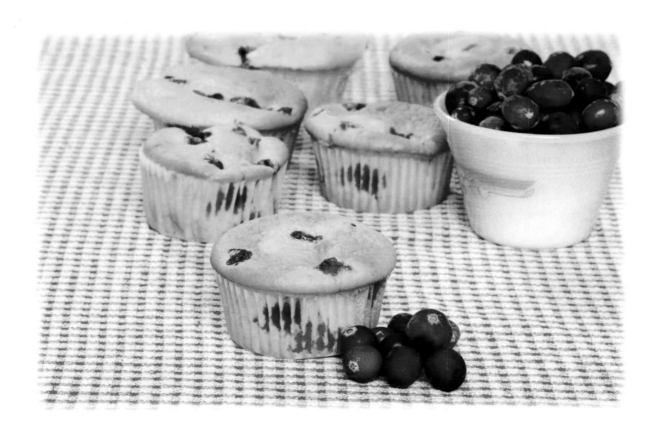

Apple and Cinnamon French Toast

Serves 12.

Time to make: 1½ hours plus eight hours refrigeration.

Ingredients:

- 3 tablespoons honey
- 3 cups zero fat milk
- 2 cups liquid egg whites
- ½ cup chopped raisins
- 1 cup dried apples (chopped)
- 1lb sliced whole wheat bread
- 1½ teaspoons vanilla extract
- 1 tablespoon confectioners' sugar
- 1½ teaspoons ground cinnamon
- ½ teaspoon ground nutmeg
- ¼ teaspoon salt

Method:

1

Whisk the honey, vanilla, salt, egg whites and milk together in a large bowl.

2

Trim the crusts off of eight slices of bread and put to one side.

3

Cut the remaining bread into 1" pieces.

4

Toss this cut bread with the cinnamon, nutmeg, raisins and dried apples in a separate bowl.

5

Coat with cooking spray a 9x13" baking pan.

6

Put the bread mixture into the pan and lay the slices without the crusts on top, trimming as necessary to fit.

7

Whisk the milk mixture again and then pour over the bread evenly.

8

Using the back of a wooden spoon press the bread down and make sure it is evenly moist.

9

Cover with some parchment paper, then wrap in foil and refrigerate for 8 to 24 hours.

10

Preheat your oven to 350F.

11

Bake the mixture for 40 minutes then uncover and cook until it has puffed up, set and is a light brown color (around 20 minutes more).

12

Let it stand for ten minutes before dusting with the confectioners' sugar and serve.

Millet Porridge

Serves: 4

Time to make: 20 minutes

Ingredients:

- **1 cup millet**
- **3 ½ cups almond milk**
- **1 pinch salt**
- **¼ cup maple syrup**
- **¼ cup chopped walnuts**
- **2 tablespoons Goji berries**

Method:

1

Combine the milk with the salt and maple syrup in a saucepan and stir in the millet.

2

Place the pan over low heat and cook it until it absorbs most of the liquid and turns creamy.

3

Stir in the Goji berries and walnuts and serve it warm or chilled.

Egg in Avocado

Serves: 2

Time to make: 25 minutes

Ingredients:

- 1 ripe avocado
- 2 eggs
- 1 pinch salt
- 1 pinch freshly ground pepper
- 1 tablespoon chopped cilantro

Method:

1

Cut the avocado in half lengthwise.

2

Remove the pit and scoop out part of the pulp.

3

Crack open the eggs and place them in each avocado half.

4

Sprinkle with salt, freshly ground pepper and chopped cilantro and bake them in the preheated oven at 375F for 15-20 minutes.

5

Serve them warm.

Vegetarian Lunches

Lunch is important to get you through the day and stop you wanting to grab snacks. Many of these lunches can be taken to work so that you can eat a healthy meal in the middle of the day and stick to your diet.

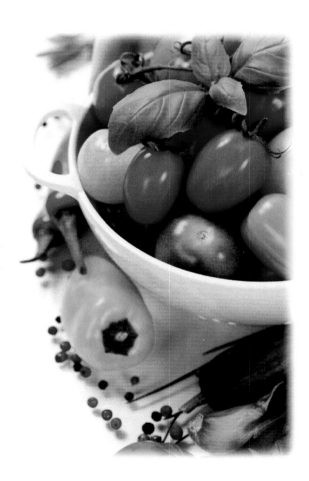

Tofu and Quinoa Salad

Serves 6.

Time to make: 35 minutes

Ingredients:

- 1 diced yellow bell pepper
- 1 cup halved grape tomatoes
- 1 cup diced cucumber
- 8oz pack of baked, smoked tofu (diced)
- 1 cup rinsed quinoa
- 2 cups water
- ¾ teaspoon salt (divided)
- 2 minced garlic cloves
- 3 tablespoons extra-virgin olive oil
- ¼ cup lemon juice
- ½ cup fresh parsley (chopped)
- ½ cup fresh mint (chopped)
- ¼ teaspoon fresh ground pepper

Method:

1

Boil the water in a saucepan with half a teaspoon of salt in it.

2

Add the quinoa and boil. Turn the heat down and simmer for 15 to 20 minutes until the water is absorbed.

3

Spread the quinoa over a baking sheet and let it cool for ten minutes.

4

Whisk the garlic, oil, lemon juice, quarter teaspoon salt and the pepper in a large bowl.

5

Add the cooled quinoa and the rest of the ingredients.

6

Toss the mixture well and serve.

Warm Squash Salad

Serves: 4

Time to make: 40 minutes

Ingredients:

- **3 cups butternut squash cubes**
- **2 tablespoons olive oil**
- **Salt, pepper to taste**
- **1 teaspoon dried oregano**
- **2 tablespoons sliced almonds**
- **2 tablespoons chopped cilantro**
- **1 tablespoon Dijon mustard**
- **2 tablespoons balsamic vinegar**
- **2 tablespoons lemon juice**
- **3 oz. feta cheese, crumbled**

Method:

1

Place the squash cubes in a baking tray and drizzle them with 2 tablespoons olive oil. Sprinkle with salt, pepper and dried oregano.

2

Bake them at 375F for 30 minutes or until they start to look caramelized.

3

Transfer them in a large bowl and stir in the sliced almonds and chopped cilantro.

4

To make the dressing, mix the mustard with the balsamic vinegar and lemon juice. Pour the dressing over the warm squash and mix gently.

5

Place the salad on a platter and top with crumbled feta before serving.

Avocado and White Bean Wrap

Serves 4.

Time to make: 25 minutes.

Ingredients:

- 1 ripened avocado
- 15oz can white beans (rinsed)
- 1 shredded carrot
- 2 cups shredded red cabbage
- whole wheat wraps or tortillas (8 to 10 inches across)
- ½ cup shredded sharp Cheddar cheese (vegetarian)
- ¼ cup chopped cilantro
- 2 tablespoons cider vinegar
- 2 tablespoons minced red onion
- 1 tablespoon canola oil
- 2 teaspoons finely chopped canned chipotle chilli
- ¼ teaspoon salt

Method:

1

Whisk the vinegar, salt, oil and chipotle chilli in a bowl.

2

Add the carrot, cabbage and cilantro and combine by tossing.

3

Mash the avocado and beans in another bowl and stir in the onion and cheese.

4

Spread ½ cup of the bean/avocado mix on to a wrap and top with around two thirds of a cup of cabbage/carrot mix. Roll up.

5

Repeat for each wrap and cut in half to serve.

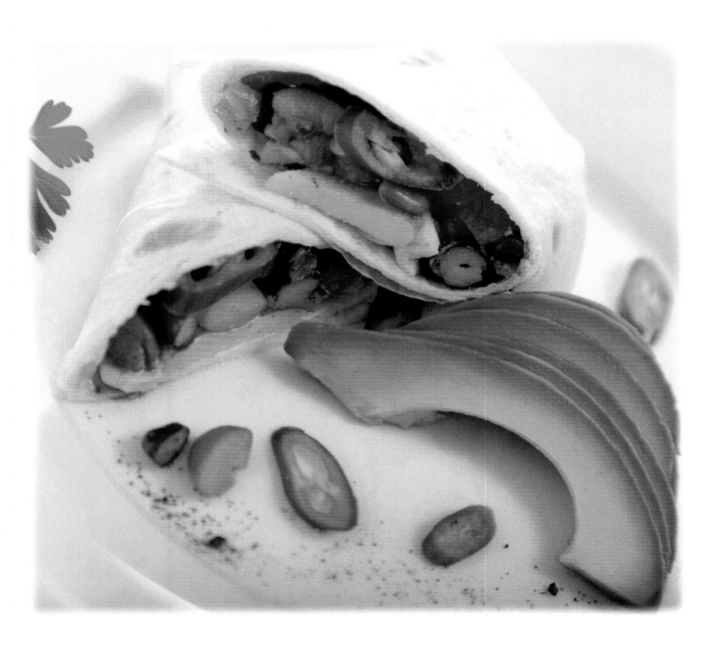

Spiced Cauliflower Patties

Serves: 8

Time to make: 40 minutes

Ingredients:

- **1 head cauliflower, cut into florets**
- **2 green onions, chopped**
- **¼ cup chopped parsley**
- **½ teaspoon cumin powder**
- **1 pinch chili flakes**
- **½ teaspoon turmeric**
- **¼ teaspoon ground coriander**
- **2 tablespoons lemon juice**
- **2 mint leaves, chopped**
- **4 tablespoons almond flour**
- **1 egg**
- **2 tablespoons olive oil**
- **Salt, pepper to taste**

Method:

1

Place the cauliflower in a food processor and pulse until ground. Transfer it into a bowl and stir in the rest of the ingredients, except the olive oil.

2

Adjust the taste with salt and pepper then form patties and place them all on a baking tray lined with parchment paper.

3

Drizzle the patties with olive oil and bake them at 350F for 20-30 minutes or until tender and golden brown.

4

Serve them simple or with a fresh salad.

Lime Roasted Tofu

Serves 4

Time to make: 1½ hours

Ingredients:

- 14pz extra firm tofu (water packed and drained)
- tablespoons toasted sesame oil
- Third of a cup of lime juice
- Third of a cup of low sodium soy sauce

Method:

1

Pat the tofu dry and cut into half inch cubes.

2

Mix the soy sauce, oil and lime juice in a shallow dish.

3

Add the tofu and gently toss, making sure it is well combined.

4

Marinate for between one and four hours in the refrigerator, stirring a couple of times.

5

Preheat your oven to 450F.

6

Remove the tofu using a slotted spoon and discard the marinade.

7

Spread the tofu out on a baking tray, ensuring the pieces are not touching.

8

Roast for about 20 minutes until golden brown, turning one.

Mediterranean Roasted Tomato Soup

Serves: 6

Time to make: 40 minutes

Ingredients:

- 1 ½ pounds ripe tomatoes
- 1 red bell pepper, cored and sliced
- 1 red onion, sliced
- garlic cloves, peeled
- 2 rosemary sprigs
- 2 tablespoons olive oil
- 2 cups vegetable stock
- Salt, pepper to taste
- 2 tablespoons chopped basil

Method:

1

Place the vegetables in a baking tray and season them with salt and pepper.

2

Drizzle them with olive oil and cook them in the preheated oven at 400F for 20 minutes or until they begin to caramelize.

3

Transfer the veggies in a pot and add in the rosemary and stock.

4

Cook another 10 minutes then puree the soup with an immersion blender.

5

Pour the soup in serving bowls and top with chopped basil before serving.

Tofu Peanut Wrap

Serves 1.

Time to make: 10 minutes

Ingredients:

- **8" whole wheat flour tortilla**
- **2oz baked seasoned tofu (sliced thinly)**
- **¼ cup red bell pepper (sliced)**
- **1 tablespoon Thai peanut sauce**
- **snow peas (thinly sliced)**

Method:

1

Spread the peanut sauce on the tortilla.

2

Place the rest of the ingredients in the middle, fold the sides over and roll up.

Barbecue Tofu Sandwich

Serves 4.

Time to make: 25 minutes

Ingredients:

- whole wheat toasted hamburger buns
- dill pickle slices
- 14oz extra firm water packed tofu (drained)
- ½ cup barbecue sauce
- 1½ cups coleslaw or shredded cabbage
- ¼ cup onion (sliced thinly)
- 2 tablespoons low fat mayo
- 1 tablespoon canola oil
- 2 teaspoons red wine vinegar
- ¼ teaspoon garlic powder
- Salt / pepper to taste

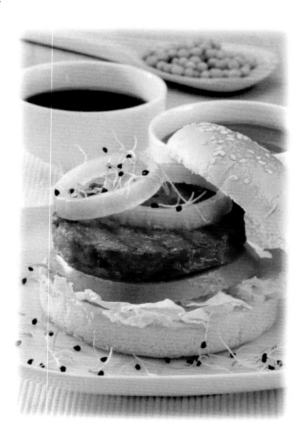

Method:

1

Put the onion in small bowl, cover it with cold water and put to one side.

2

Standing the tofu on its long side, cut it lengthwise into four slabs about ¼ thick. Pat each slice dry and sprinkle with salt.

3

Heat the oil in a non-stick pan.

4

Add the tofu slabs and cook until brown on both sides (around four minutes per side).

5

Reduce the heat and add the barbecue sauce, turning the tofu carefully to ensure it is coated on both sides.

6

Cover the pan and cook for another three minutes.

7

Whilst this is cooking, mix the mayo, vinegar, garlic powder, pepper and coleslaw in a bowl. Drain the water from the onion.

8

Place a third of a cup of coleslaw mixture on each bun, top with a slab of tofu, a slice of pickle and some slices of onion. Spread with any remaining sauce before serving.

Greek Spinach Pie

Serves: 10

Time to make: 1 hour

Ingredients:

- sheets phyllo pastry dough
- cups fresh spinach, shredded
- 1 shallot, chopped
- 2 garlic cloves, chopped
- 2 tablespoons olive oil
- 2 green onions, chopped
- ¼ cup chopped parsley
- oz. feta cheese, crumbled
- Salt, pepper to taste

Method:

1

Heat the olive oil in a large skillet. Stir in the shallot and garlic and sauté for 2 minutes.

2

Stir in the spinach and sauté for 10 minutes until softened.

3

Remove from heat and add the green onions, chopped parsley, salt and pepper.

4

Take 2 phyllo dough sheets and place them in a round cooking pan.

5

Spoon in the spinach filling and top with crumbled feta.

6

Top with the remaining phyllo dough and cook the pie in the preheated oven at 350F for 40-45 minutes or until golden brown and crisp.

7

Let it cool down before serving.

Chickpea Cilantro Salad

Serves: 4

Time to make: 15 minutes

Ingredients:

- cups canned chickpeas, rinsed and drained
- 1/3 cup chopped cilantro
- 2 ripe tomatoes, sliced
- 1 red onion, finely sliced
- 1 garlic clove, chopped
- 2 tablespoons lemon juice
- 1 tablespoon balsamic vinegar
- 2 tablespoons olive oil
- Salt, pepper to taste

Method:

1

Place the chickpeas, cilantro, tomatoes, red onion and garlic in a bowl and set aside.

2

To make the dressing for the salad, mix the lemon juice with the balsamic vinegar, olive oil, salt and pepper to taste.

3

Pour the dressing over the chickpeas and mix gently.

4

Serve the salad fresh.

Vegetable Rice Stew

Serves: 8

Time to make: 40 minutes

Ingredients:

- 1 cup brown rice
- tablespoons olive oil
- 1 shallot, finely chopped
- 2 garlic cloves, chopped
- 2 carrots, sliced
- 1 cup baby corn, sliced
- 1 cup green beans
- 1 cup green beans, chopped
- 2 cups water
- ½ cup coconut milk
- ½ teaspoon cumin powder
- 1 pinch chili powder
- tablespoons chopped cilantro
- Salt, pepper to taste

Method:

1

Heat the skillet over medium flame and stir in the shallot and garlic. Sauté for 2 minutes.

2

Stir in all the vegetables and the rice and sauté for 5 more minutes.

3

Pour in the water and coconut milk then add the cumin powder and chili.

4

Turn the heat on low and cover the skillet with a lid. Cook for 20-30 minutes until all the liquid has been absorbed and the veggies are tender.

5

Remove from heat and adjust the taste with salt and pepper then stir in the chopped cilantro.

6

Serve it warm.

Grapefruit and Cranberry Mixed Green Salad

Serves 12.

Time to make: 25 minutes

Ingredients:
- red grapefruit
- cups baby spinach
- cups torn butter lettuce
- 14oz can heart of palm (drained and cut into 1" chunks)
- Third of a cup each of toasted pine nuts and dried cranberries
- 2 tablespoons minced scallion
- 1 tablespoon white wine vinegar
- ¼ cup extra-virgin olive oil
- Salt / pepper to taste

Method:

1

Carefully remove the skin and pith from each grapefruit.

2

Holding the whole grapefruit over a bowl, cut the segments out and then cut them in half. Put these in a large salad bowl.

3

Squeeze what is left of the grapefruit (peel / pith) over a bowl to get about a quarter of a cup of grapefruit juice.

4

Whisk the scallions, vinegar and oil into the bowl with the grapefruit juice and season to taste.

5

Add the spinach, hearts of palm and lettuce to the salad bowl containing the grapefruit segments.

6

Prior to serving, toss the salad in the dressing to coat well and sprinkle the pine nuts and cranberries on top.

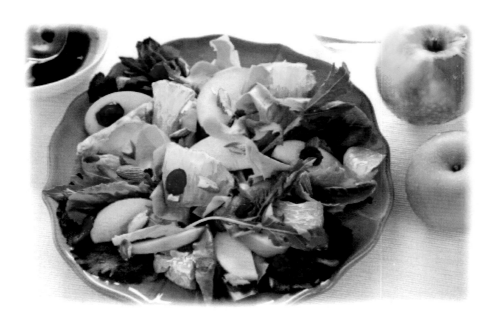

Eggplant and Portobello Sandwich

Serves 4.

Time to make: 25 minutes

Ingredients:

- slices lightly toasted whole wheat bread
- 1 tomato (sliced)
- cups arugula or spinach
- medium Portobello mushroom caps with the gills removed
- 1 eggplant (cut into ½" slices)
- ¼ cup low fat mayo
- 1 chopped garlic clove
- Olive oil cooking spray
- Salt / pepper to taste

Method:

1

Preheat your grill to a medium / high heat

2

Mash the garlic on a cutting board with the back of a spoon until it becomes a paste.

3

Mix this with the lemon juice and mayo and put to one side.

4

Coat the eggplant and mushroom caps with the cooking spray and season to taste.

5

Grill the vegetables, turning halfway through until tender and browned. This will take around 2-3 minutes per side for the eggplant and 3-4 minutes for the mushrooms.

6

When the mushrooms have cooled slightly, slice them.

7

Spread 1½ teaspoons of the garlic mayo on to each slice of bread.

8

Layer the eggplant, mushrooms, arugula and tomato slices on to four slices of bread and top with what is left of the bread.

Italian Vegetable Hoagies

Serves 4.

Time to make: 20 minutes

Ingredients:

- 14oz can artichoke hearts (rinsed and chopped coarsely)
- 1 tomato (seeded and diced)
- ¼ cup thinly sliced red onion separated out in to rings
- – 20" baguette (whole grain is preferred)
- cups romaine lettuce (shredded)
- 2 tablespoons balsamic vinegar
- 1 tablespoon extra-virgin olive oil
- 2 slices Provolone cheese
- 1 teaspoon dried oregano

Method:

1

Put the onions in a bowl and cover with cold water. Put to one side.

2

Mix the oregano, oil, tomato, vinegar and artichoke hearts in a bowl.

3

Cut the baguette into four quarters and split each quarter horizontally.

4

Pull out half the soft bread from the inside of the baguette.

.

5

Drain the onions and pat dry on kitchen towel.

6

Divide the Provolone on the bottom part of the baguette.

7

Spread the artichoke over the cheese and top with the lettuce and onion.

8

Cover with the baguette tops and serve immediately

Blue Cheese Arugula Salad

Serves: 4

Time to make: 20 minutes

Ingredients:

- cups arugula leaves
- oz. blue cheese, crumbled
- 2 ripe pears, cored and sliced
- 2 tablespoons olive oil
- 1 tablespoon Dijon mustard
- 2 tablespoons balsamic vinegar
- ¼ teaspoon dried oregano
- Salt, pepper to taste

Method:

1

Place the arugula on a platter.

2

Top with blue cheese and sliced pears and set aside while you make the dressing.

3

For the dressing, mix the olive oil with the mustard, balsamic vinegar, dried oregano, salt and pepper to taste.

4

Drizzle the dressing over the salad and serve it fresh.

Black Eye Pea Salad

Serves 6.

Time to make: 20 minutes

Ingredients:

- 14oz can black eyed peas (rinsed)
- cups cucumber (peeled and diced)
- ¾ cup red bell pepper (diced)
- ½ cup crumbled feta cheese
- ¼ cup red onion (finely chopped)
- tablespoons black olives (chopped)
- tablespoons extra-virgin olive oil
- 2 tablespoons lemon juice
- 2 teaspoons chopped oregano
- Black pepper to taste

Method:

1

Whisk the lemon juice, oregano, oil and pepper in a large bowl until it is well combined.

2

Add the rest of the ingredients and toss to thoroughly coat.

3

Server chilled or at room temperature.

Mushroom Chili

Serves:12

Time to make: 50 minutes

Ingredients:

- tablespoons olive oil
- 2 onions, chopped
- 1 red onion, finely chopped
- garlic cloves, chopped
- 1 large carrot, diced
- 2 red bell peppers, cored and chopped
- 1 green bell pepper, cored and chopped
- 1 celery stalk, chopped
- 2 cups canned diced tomatoes
- 1 cup tomato juice
- ½ cup water
- 2 cups canned black beans, drained
- 1 ½ pounds mushrooms, chopped
- ¼ teaspoon chili powder
- 1 teaspoon cumin powder
- ½ teaspoon coriander powder
- Salt, pepper to taste

Method:

1

Heat the olive oil in a large pot. Stir in the onions and garlic and sauté for 5 minutes.

2

Stir in the rest of the ingredients and cook the chili on low to medium heat for 30-40 minutes or until the liquid has reduced.

3

Adjust the taste with salt and pepper and serve it warm, topped with chopped cilantro.

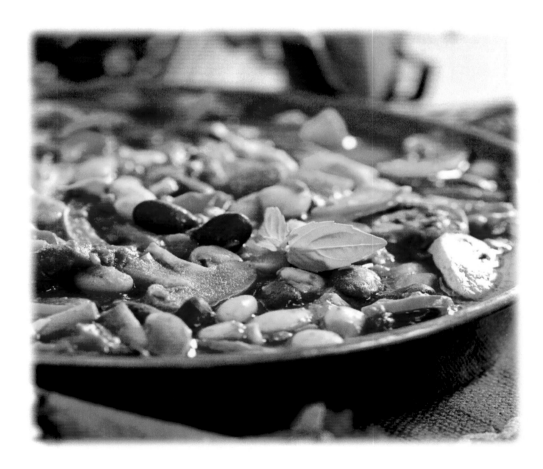

Broccoli Salad

Serves 4.

Time to make: 20 minutes

Ingredients:
- **8oz broccoli crowns (finely chopped)**
- **7oz can chickpeas (rinsed)**
- **½ cup red bell pepper (chopped)**
- **¼ cup low-fat or non-fat plain yoghurt**
- **½ cup crumbled feta cheese**
- **1 minced garlic clove**
- **1 tablespoon lemon juice**
- **¼ teaspoon freshly ground black pepper**

Method:

1

Whisk the pepper, garlic, yogurt, feta cheese and lemon juice in a bowl until thoroughly combined

2

Add the rest of the ingredients and toss to thoroughly coat.

3

Server chilled or at room temperature.

Vegetarian Dinners

Dinner is the main meal for most people and so you want a delicious meal that is filling and nutritious. This section has some great vegetarian dinners that you can cook for yourself and impress friends and family with. Many of these can be served with steamed fresh vegetables or a salad of some type to make it a complete meal.

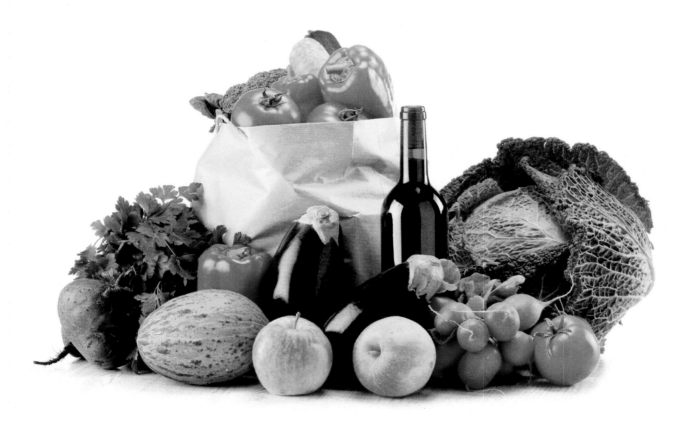

Portobello Sandwich

Serves 4 (makes 4 sandwiches).

Time to make: 25 minutes

Ingredients:

- large Portobello mushrooms with the gills and stems removed
- 1 red bell pepper (thinly sliced)
- 1 onion (sliced)
- whole wheat buns (split and toasted)
- 3oz reduced fat provolone cheese (thinly sliced)
- ¼ cup vegetable broth
- tablespoons fresh oregano (finely chopped)
- 1 tablespoon plain flour
- 1 tablespoon low sodium soy sauce
- 2 teaspoons extra-virgin olive oil
- ½ teaspoon freshly ground black pepper

Method:

1

Heat the oil in a non-stick pan over a medium to high heat.

2

Add the onion and cook for 2-3 minutes until it softens and browns.

3

Add the bell pepper, oregano, pepper and mushrooms and cook for around 7 minutes until the vegetables soften.

4

Reduce the heat and sprinkle the flour over the vegetables. Stir and ensure they are thoroughly coated.

5

Stir in the soy sauce and broth and heat to a simmer.

6

Remove from the heat and put the cheese slices over the vegetables. Cover and leave to stand for 1-2 minutes until the cheese has melted.

7

Divide the mixture into four portions. Leaving the melted cheese layer on the top, scoop each portion into a bun and serve immediately.

Zucchini Mushroom Lasagna

Serves: 9

Time to make: 1 ¼ hours

Ingredients:

- **2 zucchinis, sliced lengthwise**
- **2 pounds mushrooms**
- **1 onion, chopped**
- **2 garlic cloves, chopped**
- **2 tablespoons olive oil**
- **½ cup tomato paste**
- **2 green onions, chopped**
- **¼ cup chopped parsley**
- **2 cups tomato sauce**
- **2 cups grated mozzarella**
- **Salt, pepper to taste**

Method:

1

Heat the olive oil in a skillet and stir in the onion and garlic. Sauté for 2 minutes.

2

Mix in the mushrooms and cook 10 minutes. Add the tomato paste, salt and pepper and remove from heat.

3

To make the lasagna, take a deep dish baking pan and place a layer of zucchini slices in the pan. Top with mushroom mixture, tomato sauce and mozzarella then repeat with zucchini, sauce and cheese.

4

Finish with a layer of cheese and bake the lasagna in the preheated oven at 350F for 40-50 minutes or until soft and golden brown.

Quinoa Stuffed Squash

Serves: 6

Time to make: 1 hour

Ingredients:

- 1 small butternut squash
- garlic cloves, chopped
- 2 green onions, chopped
- cups cooked quinoa
- tablespoons chopped cilantro
- oz. feta cheese, crumbled
- 2 tablespoons chopped basil
- Salt, pepper to taste

Method:

1

Cut the squash in half and scoop out the seeds. Place the halves in a deep baking tray and set aside.

2

For the filling, combine the chopped garlic, green onions, quinoa, cilantro, chopped basil, salt and pepper.

3

Spoon the filling into both squash halves and top with crumbled feta cheese.

4

Pour 1 cup of water in the tray and cook the squash in the preheated oven at 350F for 50-60 minutes or until the squash and tender, as well as flavorful.

5

Serve it warm.

Bean Bolognese

Serves 4.

Time to cook: 40 minutes

Ingredients:
- 14oz can of chopped tomatoes
- 14oz can salad beans (rinsed)
- 1 onion (chopped)
- ½ cup carrot (chopped)
- ¼ cup celery (chopped)
- 2 tablespoons extra-virgin olive oil
- ½ cup white wine
- ¼ cup fresh parsley (chopped and divided)
- 4 garlic cloves (chopped)
- ½ cup grated Parmesan cheese
- 8oz whole wheat fettuccine
- 1 bay leaf
- ½ teaspoon salt

Method:

1

Set a large pot of water boiling.

2

Mash ½ cup of beans in a small bowl.

3

Heat the oil in a saucepan over a medium heat.

4

Add the celery, carrot, onion and salt. Cover and cook for 10 minutes until softened, stirring occasionally.

5

Add the bay leaf and garlic and cook, stirring all the time, for another 15 seconds.

6

Add the wine, turn the heat to high and boil (stirring occasionally) for 3-4 minutes until most of the liquid has gone.

7

Add the tomatoes and their juice, two tablespoons of parsley and the mashed beans.

8

Bring to a simmer, stirring occasionally, and cook for six minutes until thickened.

9

Add the whole beans and cook for another 2 minutes.

10

Meanwhile, cook the pasta until tender (about 9 minutes) and drain.

11

Divide the pasta between four bowls.

12

Discard the bay leaf and pour the sauce over the pasta.

13

Sprinkle with the cheese and the rest of the parsley.

Parmigiana Tofu

Serves 4.

Time to make: 30 minutes

Ingredients:

- **8oz mushrooms (sliced thinly)**
- **1 onion (chopped)**
- **¾ cup low sodium marinara sauce**
- **½ cup shredded low fat mozzarella cheese**
- **¼ cup plain dry breadcrumbs**
- **¼ cup grated Parmesan cheese**
- **14oz extra firm/firm water packed tofu (rinsed)**
- **tablespoons chopped fresh basil**
- **1 tablespoon plus 2 teaspoons of extra-virgin olive oil (divided)**
- **1 teaspoon Italian seasoning**
- **¼ teaspoon garlic powder**
- **¼ teaspoon salt**

Method:

1

Mix the Italian seasoning and breadcrumbs in a dish.

2

Cut the tofu into four steaks lengthwise and pat dry.

3

Sprinkle the tofu on both sides with salt and garlic powder. Then coat thoroughly in the breadcrumb mixture.

4

Heat 2 teaspoons of oil in a non-stick and add the onion. Cook for about 3 minutes until it starts to brown.

5

Add the mushrooms and cook for about four minutes until the start to brown.

6

Transfer the entire mixture to a bowl.

7

Put the tablespoon of oil in the pan and cook the tofu steaks for around 3 minutes per side until brown.

8

Turn them over and sprinkle the Parmesan cheese over the top.

9

Spoon the mushroom mixture over the top and poor the marinara sauce over this. Scatter mozzarella over the top and cook until hot and the cheese melted (around 3 minutes).

10

Sprinkle with basil and serve.

Ricotta and Spinach Stuffed Pasta Shell

Serves: 6

Time to make: 50 minutes

Ingredients:

- oz. pasta shells
- cups ricotta cheese
- 1 tablespoon lemon juice
- 2 garlic cloves, chopped
- 1 teaspoon dried oregano
- 2 tablespoons chopped basil
- cups spinach, chopped
- Salt, pepper to taste
- 2 cups tomato sauce
- ¼ cup white wine

Method:

1

In a bowl, mix the ricotta with the lemon juice, garlic, dried oregano, basil and chopped spinach. Season with salt and pepper.

2

Fill the pasta shells with the ricotta mixture and place them all in a deep dish baking pan.

3

Mix the tomato sauce with the white wine and pour it over the pasta.

4

Cook it in the preheated oven at 350F for 30-40 minutes, adding more liquid if needed.

5

Serve them warm.

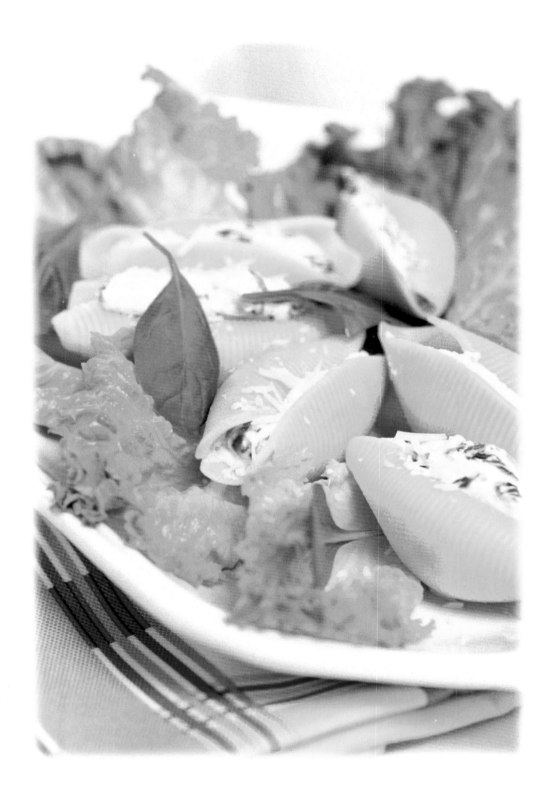

Cheese Stuffed Portobellos

Serves 4.

Time to make: 40 minutes

Ingredients:

- **Portobello mushroom caps**
- **¾ cup marinara sauce**
- **1 cup low fat ricotta cheese**
- **1 cup fresh spinach (finely chopped)**
- **tablespoons finely chopped Kalamata olives**
- **½ cup shredded Parmesan cheese (divided)**
- **½ teaspoon Italian seasoning**
- **¼ teaspoon salt**
- **¼ teaspoon freshly ground black pepper (divided)**

Method:

1

Preheat your oven to 450F.

2

Coat a baking sheet (one with a rim) with cooking spray)

3

Put the mushroom caps with the gill side up on this pan.

4

Sprinkle with salt and an eighth of a teaspoon of pepper.

5

Roast for 20-25 minutes until tender.

6

Whilst this is roasting, mast the spinach, Ricotta cheese, ¼ cup of Parmesan cheese, Italian seasoning, olives and the rest of the pepper in a bowl.

7

Warm the marinara sauce until it is hot.

8

Once the mushrooms are done, pour off any juices and return the caps to the pan.

9

Spread a tablespoon of the marinara sauce on each cap, and cover the remaining sauce to keep it warm.

10

Put a third of a cup of the ricotta mixture on to each mushroom cap and sprinkle with the rest of the Parmesan cheese.

11

Bake for another 10 minutes until hot and then serve with the rest of the marinara sauce.

Tofu Nuggets

Serves: 4

Time to make: 35 minutes

Ingredients:

- oz. firm tofu, cubed
- 1 cup vegetable stock
- tablespoons olive oil
- 2 eggs
- ½ cup all-purpose flour
- ½ cup breadcrumbs
- 1 teaspoon salt
- 2 tablespoons chopped rosemary
- ¼ teaspoon garlic powder
- 1 pinch freshly ground pepper

Method:

1

Place the tofu in a bowl and pour in the veggie stock and olive oil. Let it marinate at least 2 hour then drain the tofu cubes well.

2

Beat the eggs in a bowl and set aside.

3

In another bowl, combine the flour with the breadcrumbs, salt, rosemary, garlic powder and pepper.

4

Take each tofu cube and roll it first in egg then in the flour mixture.

5

Place all the cubes on a baking tray lined with parchment paper and bake at 400F for 20-30 minutes or until crisp and golden brown.

6

Serve them warm, simple or with a spicy sauce or a fresh salad.

Tofu Curry

Serves: 6

Time to make: 40 minutes

Ingredients:

- oz. firm tofu, cubed
- tablespoons olive oil
- 1 shallot, chopped
- 2 garlic cloves, chopped
- 1 tablespoon garam masala
- 1 tablespoon grated ginger
- ½ teaspoon turmeric
- 2 cups canned diced tomatoes
- ½ cup water
- ½ cup coconut milk
- Salt, pepper to taste

Method:

1

Heat the olive oil in a skillet. Stir in the tofu and cook them on all sides until golden brown.

2

Stir in the shallot and garlic and sauté for 2 minutes then add the garam masala, ginger and turmeric. Cook 30 seconds then add the tomatoes, water, coconut milk, salt and pepper.

3

Cover the skillet with a lid and cook for 30 minutes.

4

Serve the curry warm.

Spicy Bean Burgers

Serves 6.

Time to make: 50 minutes

Bean Burger Ingredients:
- whole wheat burger buns
- lettuce leaves
- tomato slices
- 1 minced garlic clove
- 2½ cups cooked pinto beans (drained)
- ½ cup water
- ½ cup red onion (chopped)
- ¼ cup quinoa (rinsed)
- tablespoons extra-virgin olive oil (divided)
- tablespoons fresh cilantro (chopped)
- tablespoons cornmeal plus a third of a cup for coating the burgers
- 1 teaspoon smoked paprika
- ½ teaspoon ground toasted cumin seeds
- ½ teaspoon salt

Guacamole Ingredients:
- 1 avocado (ripe)
- 1 minced garlic clove
- 2 teaspoons red onion (finely chopped)
- 2 tablespoons fresh cilantro (finely chopped)
- 1 tablespoon lemon juice
- Dash of salt and cayenne pepper (to taste)

Method:

1

Boil a pan of water, add the quinoa and bring back to the boil. Cover and simmer for about ten minutes until the water has been absorbed. Remove the cover and leave to stand.

2

Heat a tablespoon of oil on a medium heat.

3

Add the garlic and ½ cup of onion and cook for around 3 minutes, stirring occasionally.

4

Add the ground cumin, paprika and beans and mash into a smooth paste. Transfer this to a bowl and allow to cool slightly.

5

Add the quinoa, cilantro and three tablespoons of cornmeal. Season to taste and stir well.

6

Make this mixture into six burger patties and coat them with the remaining cornmeal.

7

Put them on a baking sheet and refrigerate for twenty minutes.

8

Preheat your oven to 200F.

9

Mash the avocado and stir in the rest of the guacamole ingredients.

10

Heat a tablespoon of oil in a large pan and cook three burgers in it until they are crisp and brown on both sides (around 3-4 minutes per side).

11

Transfer these to the oven to keep warm.

12

Cook the other three burgers in the same way.

13

Serve with the burgers in the buns with lettuce, tomato and guacamole.

Spiced Zucchini Boats

Serves: 6

Time to make: 40 minutes

Ingredients:

Zucchini:
- young zucchinis
- green onions, chopped
- 1 cup chopped mushrooms
- ¼ cup breadcrumbs
- 1 garlic clove, chopped
- ¼ teaspoon cumin powder
- ¼ teaspoon ground coriander
- 1 pinch chili powder
- 1 cup grated mozzarella cheese
- Salt, pepper to taste

Garlic sauce:
- garlic cloves, minced
- ½ cup low fat yogurt
- ½ cucumber, grated
- mint leaves, chopped
- Salt, pepper to taste

Method:

1

Take the zucchinis and slice them in half lengthwise. Using a teaspoon, scoop out part of the pulp and chop it finely.

2

In a bowl, combine the chopped zucchini pulp with the green onions, mushrooms, breadcrumbs, garlic, cumin powder, coriander and chili powder. Add salt and pepper to taste.

3

Spoon this mixture into each zucchini half and top with grated cheese.

4

Bake the zucchini boats in a baking tray at 350F for 30-40 minutes or until they are tender and golden brown.

5

To make the sauce, mix all the ingredients.

6

Top the zucchini with the garlic and serve warm.

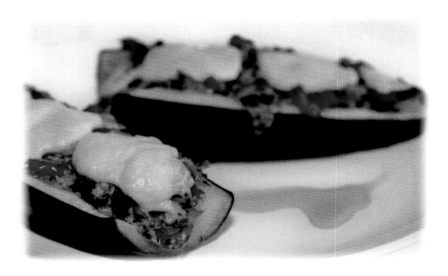

Vegetarian Taco Salad

Serves 6.

Time to make: 40 minutes

Ingredients:

- 15oz cup kidney, black or pinto beans (rinsed)
- large tomatoes (roughly chopped)
- 1½ cups corn kernels (fresh or thawed)
- 1½ cups long grain brown rice (cooked)
- 1 onion (chopped)
- cups romaine / iceberg lettuce (shredded)
- 2½ cups roughly crumbled tortilla chips
- 1 cup Pepper Jack cheese (shredded)
- ½ cup fresh cilantro (chopped)
- Third of a cup of salsa
- 2 tablespoons extra-virgin olive oil
- 1 tablespoon chilli powder
- 1½ teaspoons dried oregano (divided)
- ¼ teaspoon salt
- Lime wedges to serve

Method:

1

Heat the oil in a non-stick pan.

2

Cook the onion for around five minutes until it starts to brown.

3

Add one chopped tomato, beans, rice, chilli powder, salt and a teaspoon of oregano to the pan.

4

Cook for five minutes, stirring regularly.

5

Remove the pan from the heat and allow to cool slightly.

6

Combine the rest of the tomatoes with the salsa, cilantro and remaining oregano in a bowl.

7

Toss the lettuce together with two thirds of a cup of cheese, half the fresh salsa and the bean mixture.

8

Sprinkle the tortilla chips and the rest of the cheese over the mixture.

9

Serve with lime wedges and fresh salsa.

Black Bean Croquettes

Serves 4.

Time to make: 45 minutes

Ingredients:

- x 15oz cans of black beans (rinsed)
- 1 avocado (diced)
- 2 cups tomatoes (finely chopped)
- 2 scallions (sliced)
- ¼ cup fresh cilantro (chopped)
- 1 cup corn kernels (fresh or thawed)
- ¼ cup plus a third of a cup dry breadcrumbs (divided)
- 1 tablespoon extra-virgin olive oil
- 1 teaspoon ground cumin
- 1 teaspoon chilli powder (divided)

Method:

1

Preheat your oven to 425F and coat a baking tray with cooking oil spray.

2

Mash the cumin and black beans together until there are no whole beans left.

3

Stir in the corn kernels and the ¼ cup of breadcrumbs.

4

In a separate bowl, mix the cilantro, scallions, tomatoes, ½ teaspoon of chilli powder and salt.

5

Stir one cup of this mixture into the black bean mixture.

6

Mix the rest of the breadcrumbs together with the oil and ½ teaspoon of chilli powder until the breadcrumbs are coated with oil.

7

Divide this mixture into eight bowls, each about half a cup in size.

8

Lightly press each ball into the breadcrumbs, ensuring it is well coated and place on the baking sheet.

9

Bake until the breadcrumbs are golden brown, which will take around 20 minutes.

10

Stir the avocado into the tomato mixture and serve the salsa on the side.

Barley Risotto

Serves 6.

Time to make: 3 to 4 hours

Ingredients:

- 1 large fennel bulb (cored and diced)
- tablespoons chopped fennel fronds
- 2 teaspoons fennel seeds
- 1 carrot (finely chopped)
- 1 shallot (finely chopped)
- 2 garlic cloves (minced)
- 1 cup pearl barley
- cups vegetable broth
- 2 cups French cut green beans (frozen are fine)
- ½ cup Parmesan cheese (grated)
- 1 – 1½ cups water (divided)
- Third of a cup dry white wine
- Third of a cup black olives (coarsely chopped)
- 1 tablespoon lemon zest

Method:

1

Coat your slow cooker with cooking spray (minimum of 4 quart size).

2

Carefully crush the fennel seeds using the bottom of a saucepan.

3

Mix the diced fennel together with the barley, crushed fennel seeds, shallot, carrots and garlic into the slow cooker.

4

Add the vegetable broth, wine and a cup of water and stir well.

5

Cover and cook until the barley is tender but chewy (between 2½ and 3½ hours depending on the setting).

6

Before serving, cook the green beans and drain.

7

Turn off the slow cooker and stir in the Parmesan, olive, lemon zest and green beans. Season with pepper to taste.

8

If the mixture is too dry, heat the remaining half a cup of water and stir it in.

9

Serve sprinkled with the fennel fronds.

Chickpea Burgers

Serves 4.

Time to make: 25 minutes

Ingredients:

- 19oz can chickpeas (rinsed)
- 1 egg
- scallions (trimmed and sliced)
- whole wheat pitas (halved and warmed)
- 2 tablespoons flour
- 2 tablespoons extra-virgin olive oil
- 1 tablespoon chopped oregano
- ½ teaspoon ground cumin
- ¼ teaspoon salt

Tahini Ingredients:

- ½ cup low fat or no fat plain yogurt
- Third of a cup of chopped flat leaf parsley
- tablespoons Tahiti
- 1 tablespoon lemon juice
- ½ teaspoon salt

Method:

1

Put the egg, flour, scallions, chickpeas, cumin, oregano and salt into a food processor.

2

Pulse, stopping occasionally to scrape the mixture off the sides, until it is a coarse, moist mixture that holds together when pressed.

3

Form the mixture into four patties.

4

Heat the oil in a non-stick pan.

5

Cook the patties for around five minutes until they turn golden and begin to crisp.

6

Flip them carefully and cook for another 3 to 4 minutes until brown.

7

Mix the tahini, lemon juice, parsley, yogurt and salt in a bowl and mix.

8

Divide the patties between the pitas and serve with your sauce.

Sweet Potato Pasta

Serves 4.

Time to make: 30 minutes

Ingredients:

- cups sweet potato (shredded and peeled)
- 1 red bell pepper (thinly sliced)
- garlic cloves (minced)
- 8oz whole wheat angel hair pasta
- 1 cup plum tomatoes (diced)
- ½ cup water
- ½ cup goat cheese (crumbled)
- tablespoons extra-virgin olive oil (divided)
- 2 tablespoons fresh parsley (chopped)
- 1 tablespoon fresh tarragon (chopped)
- 1 tablespoon white wine vinegar
- ¾ teaspoon salt

Method:

1

Boil a large pan of water and cook the pasta for around five minutes until tender.

2

Cook the garlic in a tablespoon of oil in a large pan for 3 to 5 minutes until fragrant and sizzling.

3

Add the tomatoes, sweet potato, bell pepper and water and cook for another 5 to 7 minutes until the pepper is tender.

4

Remove from the heat, cover and keep warm.

5

Drain the pasta, keeping half a cup of the water.

6

Put the pasta back in the pot and add the vegetable mixture together with the white wine vinegar, salt, cheese, oil, tarragon and parsley.

7

Toss it well to combine and add the reserved pasta water a tablespoon or two at a time until you get the desired consistency.

Why Microwaving Food Is Bad For You

In modern society it is so tempting to microwave food; it's quick and convenient and saves time and effort. However, whilst you may be freezing healthy food and eating healthy food, when you zap your food in the microwave it comes out much less healthy than when you put it in. More and more people now are avoiding their microwave ovens because of the health concerns associated with their use.

When you microwave food it strips away the nutrients in the food. Your nice healthy plate of food becomes dead, as the microwaves change the molecular structure of your food. The best way to cook vegetables so that they retain the maximum amount of nutrients is to steam them.

If you microwave any food that contains vitamin B-12 then it is destroyed by the radiation. Studies have shown that around 40% of the B-12 is lost just by microwaving the food. This means that if you are microwaving foods that contain B-12 you are reducing your intake significantly by doing so.

To give you an idea of just how bad microwaves are, scientists strongly advise against microwaving breast milk because it causes E-coli bacteria to grow at eighteen times the rate of non-microwaved breast milk.

You may have heard warnings that you should not microwave food wrapped or contained in plastic. These warnings were so severe that Russia issued a health warning on microwave ovens. The toxins from plastic leak out into your food during the microwaving process and then are absorbed into your body where they have been linked with serious diseases such as cancer.

Microwaved food seems to also change your blood with studies showing people who eat microwaved food have decreased levels of red blood cells and increased white blood cells. Upsetting the balance of your body is never a good idea for your health.

Not only that, but the frequency of the radiation produced by a microwave oven affects your heart rate and your heart rate variability. Whilst it is considered "safe" according to federal guidelines, if you have any heart problems then it is only going to make it worse.

Whilst a microwave is convenient in that it makes it very quick for you to make food, the health risks offset the benefits. As a vegetarian you will want to buy a steamer, cook your vegetables in that and make lots of delicious fresh food using the recipes detailed in this book. When you realize how different and nice non-microwaved food tastes you will never look back.

Exercise And The Vegetarian

A lot of people feel that if they are eating a vegetarian or vegan diet then they can't exercise. This is a myth and many athletes are vegetarian and successful at their sport. You need to be more careful as a vegetarian to ensure you get sufficient amounts of protein, zinc, B12 and iron which is necessary for your athletic performance.

The current recommendation from the American College of Sports Medicine is that a strength athlete needs between 0.5 and 0.8g of protein per pound of body weight. As a vegetarian you can easily get plenty of protein from low fat dairy, tofu, vegetable proteins and other protein rich plant sources. To give you an idea, here are some vegetarian friendly foods and their protein levels.

8oz Milk - 8g protein
3oz Tofu – 15g protein
8oz Yogurt – 8g protein
3oz cheese – 21g protein
2 Tablespoons peanut butter – 8g protein

So you can see that it is easy to get protein from vegetarian sources.

You also need to get heme-iron, which is an easy to absorb form of iron. This is important to all athletes, particular for women, and can be obtained from leafy green vegetables, wholegrain cereals, lentils, figs and kidney beans.

Vitamin C is also important as it helps you to absorb iron and is found in lots of different fresh fruits and vegetables. Having a good combination of fruit and vegetables in your diet will ensure that you get plenty of this important vegetable. Orange juice and other citrus fruits are well known to be high in Vitamin C.

Vitamin B12 is the nutrient most commonly missing from a vegetarian diet as it is found in animal products. You only need around 2.4 micrograms every day which you can get from foods fortified with B12, vitamin supplements or from eggs, milk, yoghurt and cheese if you eat enough of them.

Foods such as whole grains, coffee, bran and spinach affect the absorption of iron by your body and if you are consuming these you need to up your vitamin C intake in order to offset the effect they have.

Dietary supplements are not to be used to offset a poor diet but they are helpful in preventing deficiencies, particularly if you are exercising a lot. If you are incorporating exercise into your life, which you should do for the health and weight benefits, then you may need pay particular attention to your diet and supplement what you eat as necessary to ensure you are receiving all the nutrients you need.

Transitioning To The Vegetarian Diet

When it comes to transitioning to this diet you need to make sure you have good solid reasons for why you are doing it. Knowing that you are becoming vegetarian in order to lose weight and be healthier is a big motivation for you and will help make switching your diet easy for you.

During the transition you need to make your meals interesting and tasty because it will encourage you to stick to the diet. There are some great recipes in this book to get you started and don't worry if you feel you can't cook; it's easier than it looks!

Try different recipes every week and soon you will have a good list of meals that you enjoy cooking and eating. You can also try the meals you like but with a meat substitute. So if you love lasagne, try making one but without the meat; use a textured vegetable (TVP) protein instead. Most meat eaters won't be able to taste the difference!

If you are not going to go cold turkey then start by cutting red meat from your diet and eat a couple of vegetarian meals per week. Gradually increase the number of vegetarian meals you eat and then cut out poultry and pork, and keep increasing the amount of vegetarian meals you are eating. Finally, cut out seafood and then you should be a full time vegetarian.

You need to think about what type of vegetarian you are going to be. Are you going to continue eating both dairy and eggs? One or the other? Neither? It is up to you, though many people like the dairy (in moderation) and eggs because they are a good source of calcium, Omega-3 and other essential vitamins.

Look at the foods that you regularly eat and see which ones are vegetarian and which ones are not. For those that are not, start clearing them out and replacing them with vegetarian friendly versions. Start to stock your cupboards with these foods and pay attention to what you are eating during the day and make sure it is all vegetarian.

Whilst you can go cold turkey and give up meat all at once, for many people that is just too much. However, if you can then do it because it can be an easy way to become vegetarian, as you are not still eating meat and your body can start to clear the residues of meat out of your system.

You will want to let friends and family know about your choice too because you don't want them to make you food you then either have to reject it or force yourself to eat it so you don't hurt their feelings. Often you will get support from them and they will be encouraging to you. However, on occasion there will be resistance from them. Just don't try to force them to become vegetarian and preach to them, just explain you have made a lifestyle choice for your health.

Being vegetarian isn't like retreating into a mountain top cave to become a hermit. It is meant to be a fun diet and something you can enjoy, so make it so! Be creative with your meals, experiment with flavors, spices and dressings (all vegetarian of course) and make yourself interesting food! It will help make the transition to the new diet much easier for you.

In your early months as a vegetarian you will need to plan ahead in what you are cooking, where you are eating and so on. You may find that you need to take snacks with you or prepare meals in advance. This is one way of avoiding temptation and making sure you have food you can eat when you need it.

Transitioning to the vegetarian diet will depend on your personality and your lifestyle. However you choose to do it though, make sure you set realistic goals and you stick to them!

Eating Out On The Vegetarian Diet

As with any diet, eating out can be a bit of trial, though on the vegetarian diet it is often less so. Dieters often feel excluded from meals out, but almost every restaurant has vegetarian options and even if they don't you can still find something to eat from the menu with a bit of creativity on your part (and sometimes on the chef's too).

If you can't see any main course vegetarian meals then you can either ask that the meat components are removed from a main meal or you can build a meal from the starters. In a lot of restaurants you can put together a delicious meal from these smaller dishes and keep it low fat and healthy too!

If you go to the more upmarket restaurants then you can ask the chef to prepare you a vegetarian dish. Most will be more than happy to do so and show off their skills to you. Just talk nicely to your waiter and they will be happy to help you, though failing that you can call ahead and arrange for something to be prepared for you.

Salad bars, soups (meat free of course), baked potatoes and starters can all be combined to make for a delicious meal for you, no matter where you are eating out. Even fast food restaurants now offer vegetarian alternatives, in most cases, and often a meat free salad too.

The hard part of becoming a vegetarian can be eating at the homes of friends or family; sometimes someone just won't accept that you don't eat meat. Maybe they think you are being unhealthy or maybe they just can't imagine life without meat, but they often will actively sabotage your efforts to be a vegetarian.

However, if you don't inform them of your vegetarianism then they can't be blamed for not being psychic and preparing you something in advance. Just explain to them that you have made a lifestyle choice and if they start arguing ask them to respect your decisions. In most cases they will be happy with it, but in some areas of the world and in some states it can be harder to be a vegetarian.

Eating out as a vegetarian isn't as hard as on other diets, there are plenty of different types of food you can eat. Sometimes you will have to be more creative than others, but generally you will get by, get the healthy option and help yourself to lose weight.

Tips For Weight Loss Success

Whilst the vegetarian diet will help you to lose weight, just cutting out meat isn't enough; you need to follow some basic weight loss strategies to ensure you lose weight. This chapter contains some tips that will help you to get rid of that weight quickly.

Every time you go to put food in your mouth you need a table, plate and a chair. This rule is very simple but it ensures you are not sneaking food, snacking or getting a thousand plus calories from a fast food meal. This simple rule keeps you aware of what you are eating and helps you to keep your calorie intake down; you also find you eat less because you are consciously aware of what you are eating.

Every diet, including this one requires willpower and you will have to learn to exercise it and build it up! Lack of willpower is probably the number one cause of breaking a diet and it has nothing to do with genetics, it's a learned response! Willpower tends to wane when you are tired and run down, so plan your diet around this fact. If you know when you get in from work you will be tired and hungry, prepare your meals in advance so you just have to heat them up.

You also need to be realistic with your weight loss plans. You aren't likely to lose ten pounds in a week and you will struggle to lose weight if you don't exercise and reduce your calorie intake. You will find that after a couple of weeks you will hit a plateau and you need to break through it. Aim to lose two pounds a week – that's very realistic and achievable as well as being a healthy amount of weight to lose; losing too much weight too quickly is actually harmful to your body. Also remember that as you age it becomes easier to put on weight and harder to lose it!

Look at your friends as well – are they people who encourage you to eat and are unhealthy people themselves? If they are then you may need to re-think your social circle as you can find that your willpower is pushed to breaking point by them. Find some healthy groups of friends and start hanging out with them; it will help to make you even healthier!

When you go shopping, avoid the aisles where the unhealthy food lurks. Before you go to the checkout, check the contents of your cart and remove the unhealthy products that have "fallen" in to it. These unhealthy snacks contribute to weight gain and by just taking a moment to review your shopping choices you will buy healthier food. Also, avoid shopping when you are hungry; eat before you shop because otherwise you will be buying all sorts of snack foods because you hungry!

Don't eat because of something. If you go to a ball game, don't eat a hotdog; if you go to the movies, skip the popcorn and soda. Teach yourself that you only eat when you are hungry and it will contribute significantly to you losing weight.

Most of us spend all day, every day sitting down and living a sedentary lifestyle that is highly effective in helping us put on weight. Get a step counter and set yourself targets for walking 10,000 or 15,000 steps a day! Instead of emailing a colleague at work, walk over to them; take the stairs not the elevator; park further away from the office door. All of this helps you to burn more calories and get fitter. Combine this with a visit to the gym and you'll be helping your health and weight loss progress nicely.

Some people also eat because of stress, which is a habit you need to get out of as doing so can lead to significant weight loss. You may think you can put off your diet until a time when you have no stress, but that is never going to happen! Learning to cope with stress without food is vital because otherwise you will struggle to lose weight. Learn positive coping methods such as meditation, yoga and so on; all of which will help you to cope with stress.

Conclusion

If you are keen to lose weight and to improve your health then the vegetarian diet is for you. With more and more people concerned about the quality of meat and the health implications of eating it, this is an ideal diet which will benefit you in many different ways.

Vegetarianism has been proven to be beneficial to your health, helping you to live longer and healthier. Many vegans and vegetarians do not experience heart complaints or high cholesterol until much later in life because of the lower fat, higher vegetable diet.

You have learnt a lot about the vegetarian diet in this book and now you need to start transitioning to this diet. Whether you go cold turkey or gradually decrease the amount of meat is up to you; only you will know what is best for your body. However, don't drag it out too long, have a definite plan and stick to it.

As you become a vegetarian you will notice that you feel different and better. The heavy feeling of eating a meal will go and you will feel lighter because your body does not have to expend so much energy digesting food. Red meat is known to sit in your intestine for weeks, which obviously won't happen on this diet as you don't eat red meat.

This book has given you some ideas for some delicious meals that you can cook to get you started on the vegetarian diet, many of which are surprisingly simple to make! You may think that being a vegetarian is difficult but actually today it is easier than ever with many different meat substitutes and more and more people turning to this diet every day.

Now it is time to make that move to vegetarianism and to benefit from losing weight and improving your health. Just by cutting out meat you can lose a pound or sometimes more each week; cut down on the junk food too and you'll find the weight just dropping off you. It's an easy diet to follow and one that makes it easy for you to eat out as well.

Enjoying following the vegetarian diet and benefiting from it. It's a fantastic diet that is going to make a huge difference in your life and help you to get to the weight you want.

Made in the USA
Middletown, DE
20 March 2018